MW01089992

Spinal Stenosis and Back Pain Relief Treatments Reviewed

36 Pain Relief Procedures, Exercises, Alternatives, Gadgets, and Ointments Reviewed by a Spinal Stenosis Sufferer

By
Gary Hennerberg

Spinal Stenosis and Back Pain Relief Treatments Reviewed
Pain Relief Procedures, Exercises, Alternatives, Gadgets, and
Ointments
Reviewed by a Spinal Stenosis Sufferer

© 2018 Gary Hennerberg

Published by Hennerberg Group, Inc.

ISBN: 978-1-79543-589-5

Notice

Gary Hennerberg (hereafter referred to as the "Author") is providing *Spinal Stenosis and Back Pain Relief Treatments Reviewed* (hereafter referred to as the "Book") and its contents on an "as is" basis and makes no representations or warranties of any kind with respect to this Book or its contents. The Author disclaims all such representations and warranties, including, for example, warranties of merchantability and fitness for a particular purpose. In addition, the Author does not represent or warrant that the information accessible via this Book is complete or current.

The statements made about products and services have not been evaluated by the U.S. Food and Drug Administration. They are not intended to diagnose, treat, cure, or prevent any condition or disease. Please consult with your own physician or healthcare specialist regarding the reviews made in this Book.

Except as specifically stated in this Book, the author will not be liable for damages arising out of or in connection with the use of this Book. This is a comprehensive limitation of liability that applies to all damages of any kind, including (without limitation) compensatory damages; direct, indirect, or consequential damages; loss of income, or profit; loss of or damage to property; and claims of third parties.

This Book provides content related to topics about back pain relief. As such, use of this Book implies your acceptance of the terms described herein.

You understand that a private citizen, without any professional training in the medical, health, or nutritional field, authored this Book. You understand that this Book is provided to you without a health examination and without prior discussion of your health condition. You understand that in no way will this Book provide medical advice and that no medical advice is contained in this Book.

You understand that this Book is not intended as a substitute for consultation with a licensed healthcare practitioner, such as your physician. Before you begin any health modification program, or change your lifestyle in any way, you should consult your physician or other licensed healthcare practitioner to ensure that you are in good health and that the advice contained in this Book will not harm you.

Table of Contents

Introduction

Introduction

For the record: I am not trained in medicine, nursing, physical therapy, chiropractic, or any of the treatments I'm reviewing.

I'm a back pain sufferer, diagnosed with spinal stenosis, and this short book discusses three dozen things that I have tried in recent years. Some I still use today. Others I've stopped using after I didn't find they helped me.

Everyone is different. What worked for me may not work for you.

Over the years, I've come to know how to spot someone with back pain a mile away. It's the way a person holds their shoulders, their back, their gait, and that look of agony on their face.

I was first diagnosed with spinal stenosis in 2010. I was in pain and couldn't understand why it wouldn't go away. The pain was getting worse and I was desperate for relief. I met with a surgeon who told me the only relief would come from spinal fusion surgery. Soon after the appointment with the physician, I decided to have spinal fusion surgery. I had five years of more good days than bad days.

But then the stenosis came back in July 2015, spreading to the spinal column both above and below where I had the surgery. It was discouraging, to say the least.

Over the years, I've tried some 36 medical procedures, alternative approaches, exercise, prescriptions, over-the-counter pills, creams, and more.

The bad news: I conclude there is apparently no fix that will permanently eliminate my spinal stenosis.

The good news: I've learned by trial and error that spinal stenosis can be managed.

But with managing spinal stenosis, you must accept that there will be good days and bad days. My goal is to have more good days than bad days, and to celebrate the good days (without overdoing it and paying for it the next day).

Millions deal with back pain caused by spinal stenosis. Every day, people get MRIs and are told that they have spinal stenosis.

The Mayo Clinic says, "*Spinal stenosis is a narrowing of the spaces within your spine, which can put pressure on the nerves that travel through the spine. Spinal stenosis occurs most often in the lower back and the neck.*"

The American Academy of Orthopedic Surgeons estimates that spinal stenosis affects 8 to 11 percent of the population, mostly in people over the age of 50. So if we look at just the Baby Boomer generation of about 75 million people, this suggests there are could be 6-to-8 million people living with this condition in the U.S. My "guestimate" of the daily number of people who are either diagnosed, or realize something isn't right with their back, is about 1,000 people every day.

If you're among those who have been told that you have spinal stenosis, chances are you're researching treatments.

And that's what this short book is about: those dozens of treatments I've personally tried. There are others still out there that may help, but I believe this list covers most that are available and accessible. Many of these options are available about anywhere. But several of these you'll only find in major urban areas.

Since 2010, I've spent tens of thousands of dollars on treatments. Some help. Many don't and are a waste of time and money. With medical care costs skyrocketing, and most of us dealing with high insurance deductibles or co-pays, you need to be smart about what you try and spend your money on.

The fact is that I spend hundreds of dollars monthly to manage my back pain. I'm not pleased about it, and if you're in the same situation, surely you can't be pleased about it either.

Spinal stenosis has drained a lot of my money. I resent that sometimes. But as I see it, I can either invest the money in procedures that help me so I can continue working and physically enjoy my life most days, or be miserable and not terribly productive most—if not all—days.

It's my hope you can find something within these pages that you can try that will give you some degree of relief.

1. Physical Therapy

I begin my discussion with PT because it's likely one of the first recommendations you'll get from a physician. I've been through PT on three occasions: (1) after my first bout of pain in 2010, (2) post-shoulder rotator cuff surgery, and (3) post-spinal fusion surgery (more about spinal fusion surgery later).

I have a lot of good to say about post-surgery PT. But to help manage day-to-day spinal stenosis pain, I didn't feel that physical therapy helped me.

I have only good things to say about the many therapists I've worked with over the years that have helped me post-surgery. They are why I regained virtually all mobility after my rotator cuff surgery and helped me recover use of muscles after my spinal fusion surgery.

So, if your physician prescribes physical therapy, it will likely be suggested that you try a specific number of PT visits over a few weeks.

Cost:

Depending upon your insurance or Medicare coverage, you may have to make co-payments. I found that my out-of-pocket (before meeting a sky-high deductible) was around $80 per visit. The doctor's orders can call for three visits weekly for six weeks. That's 18 appointments, and at $80 per visit, for a total of $1,440.

Bottom line:

Try it. But be mindful if it's helping you or not.

2. Epidural Steroid Injection

In addition to physical therapy, there's a good chance a physician will recommend an epidural steroid injection.

Over the course of six years, I've probably had nearly a dozen of these procedures. I've experienced relief, even if only for a few weeks. Back in 2010, I had an injection just days before a planned family vacation, which enabled me to enjoy my vacation much more.

You may find that an injection or two can help you return to normal. I have a friend who has to get one of these every few years and it helps him for years instead of just months. But he doesn't have spinal stenosis. Most people I've spoken with have the same result that I have: it works for a short time and you have to keep repeating it.

If you have an important event in your life coming up where you want pain relief, then go for it. But you should know it's an expensive procedure. If insurance picks up most of the cost, great. If you have a high deductible, as most people do these days, and you're going to have to pay for it all, make sure to ask both the doctor and facility your out-of-pocket cost. Then talk to your insurance company prior to the procedure to see what they'll negotiate as a lower cost so you'll know in advance what your financial responsibilities will be to make an informed financial decision.

All that said, I found that steroids wreak havoc on my sleep and mood. If you get into a cycle of repeated injections (as I did from 2015–2016), you might notice odd feelings and feeling a bit "off." Remember, we're talking steroids. I was advised I could only have a three-or-so of these annually. The effect of one would wear off before I was eligible for the next.

Cost:

Thousands of dollars.

Bottom line:

Consider this procedure if a) you are in terrible pain, b) you can afford it, and c) you have the strength to not let yourself become addicted. I don't plan to get an epidural spinal injection again, unless my stenosis declines so much that it becomes close to a final option.

3. Facet Joint Injection

Facet joints are small joints at each segment of the spine that provide stability and help guide motion. A cervical, thoracic or lumbar facet joint injection involves injecting a small amount of local anesthetic (numbing agent) and/or steroid medication, which can anesthetize the facet joints and block the pain.

I had to have a test, of sorts, a few days before the actual full procedure to see if it would work. I was (temporarily) amazed. When my wife and I went on a walk a few hours later, I remarked how I was able to take longer strides and walk faster. I felt great!

As in the case of the epidural steroid injection, if you have an event coming up where you just don't want the distraction and limitation of constant pain, this one could help.

But it only lasts a few weeks. And you'll want to check with your health insurance carrier to see how frequently you can get this type of injection. And be informed about your responsibility of paying for it before committing.

Cost:

Like other medical procedures, it costs thousands of dollars. Only you (and your insurance coverage) can determine if the value is there for you.

Bottom line:

Like the epidural steroid injection, consider this procedure if you are in terrible pain and can afford it.

4. Rhizotomy

Rhizotomy is a surgical procedure to sever nerve roots in the spinal cord. The procedure can relieve chronic back pain and muscle spasms. For spinal joint pain, a facet rhizotomy may provide lasting low back pain relief by disabling the sensory nerve at the facet joint.

With this procedure, a needle with a probe is inserted just outside the joint. The probe is then heated with radio waves and applied to the sensory nerve to the joint in order to disable the nerve. Theoretically, by deadening the sensory nerve to the facet joint, a facet rhizotomy can prevent pain signals from getting to the brain.

Research suggests it works for about half of patients. And it's multiple times the cost of the injection procedures previously discussed.

I was told it usually works for six to twelve months, hence why I decided to try it. But for me, after four months it had worn off. But the four months were good ones.

Cost:

After my insurance company adjusted the nearly $14,000 billed cost, between insurance and my co-pay, my cost was around $7,000, or about $60 a day for the four-month duration. Another consideration: my insurance company allowed only a limited number of various procedures (epidural spinal injections, facet joint injection and rhizotomies) each year.

Bottom line:

I did get relief from the rhizotomy. But the cost is high, and the inability to repeat it soon was discouraging.

5. Platelet Rich Plasma Regenerative Treatment

Platelet Rich Plasma (PRP) treatments are a new development in regenerative therapies. Platelets are tiny cells that contain thousands of growth factors that are critical to healing. They are the body's primary source of bioactive tissue growth factors. These compounds control and regulate your natural healing process in response to degenerative changes.

By concentrating the platelets and injecting them into the site of the problem, the healing process can stimulate stem cells.

For some individuals, stem cell therapy may be possible (more about stem cells in Additional Options).

In the case of the PRP procedure I experienced, the medical office drew blood from my arm (about half a pint). The blood was sent to a lab where a device concentrated the platelets up to 40 times, resulting in "Super Concentrated Platelets." After about four hours, my own blood, after having the platelets concentrated, was injected into my low back. There were three points of injection, each going in about two inches. I was able to watch the needle movement in my back. In the office where I went, there was no anesthesia or pain killers administered. It was very painful, but the injection only took about 15 minutes.

I was told it could take 3 to 5 weeks before I would feel relief, but after just a few days I sensed the pain had subsided. Even months after the procedure, I could tell the edge was taken off the pain. While there is still some ache, I realize there are moments where I'm completely pain-free. Sitting for longer periods (such as sitting at a desk or driving long distances) is less painful than it was prior to this procedure.

Cost:

My procedure cost $1,200. It was not covered by insurance and completely out-of-pocket.

Bottom line:

I will repeat this procedure every few months as needed. If you consider PRP, do your homework. I have learned that not every PRP procedure is the same. Some will draw blood and rather than process the blood in a lab, will spin it in a bedside centrifuge. Ask what the concentration will be of your blood. Some providers will concentrate it five times. Others, such as the facility I used, concentrate the blood up to 40 times. Higher, as I understand it, is better.

6. Spinal Fusion Surgery

After dealing with back pain for months back in 2010, and exhausting other medical options such as physical therapy and injections, it came to an appointment with a back surgeon. He took one look at my MRI and said the only option was surgery.

So I did it. My L4 and L5 lumbar vertebrae were fused, and for the rest of my life I'll have titanium screws and rods in my back. Actually, I was happy with it for five years until the narrowing of the spaces within my spine returned—this time in the L3 mostly in the area above the fusion. If I had realized that was likely to happen, I may have had second thoughts about doing the surgery.

Make no mistake: this is a major surgery. I was hospitalized for three days. The next ten days at home were tough. After about two weeks, I was able to work a couple of hours daily, and slowly got back to work full time. It took about 6-8 weeks before I had mostly recovered. The pain killers were tough to wean myself from (more about that in the section about prescription medications). Then, the surgery was followed with more physical therapy.

I had five pretty good years after the surgery. I experienced more good days than bad days.

Cost:

Ridiculously expensive. In 2010, the combined bills approached a quarter of a million dollars. Insurance negotiated it way down, and in 2010, my insurance deductible wasn't as outrageously high as it is now. Since you're bound to meet your deductible immediately, you should know what the maximum out-of-pocket cost you'll incur so you're financially informed.

Bottom line:

Knowing what I did in 2010, it was the right decision for me then. But now that I've found alternatives, I probably would first have tried the alternatives for a year or more to see if I had any progress with those.

7. NSAIDs, Opioids, and Prescription Medications

An NSAID (Nonsteroidal Anti-inflammatory Drug) that I took in 1990 for back pain, 20 years before the spinal stenosis diagnosis, nearly killed me. The medication worked to substantially reduce pain. But it ate holes in my stomach. I had multiple blood transfusions and, ultimately, emergency surgery in the wee hours of a Sunday morning.

I nearly died. The doctors told me that to have waited any longer for the surgery would have risked vital organs shutting down. So today I have about an 8" scar on my abdomen where they cut me open to sew the holes in my stomach together. I was hospitalized for nearly two weeks. The day after I was discharged I was back at the ER, only to find out that the holes reappeared. I spent another week in the hospital. The drug was that strong.

As you can understand, NSAIDs scare the living daylights out of me.

Years later, after a couple of surgeries, I have taken other pain killers. In those cases, I took opioid pain medication. If you've had surgery, you understand why you need an opioid pain killer of such high strength.

After my spinal fusion in 2010, I was on one of those opioids for many days. It took time to wean myself from it. I can see why they are addictive. During the three days I chose to ease off and discontinue them, I felt like I had the flu (I later read that flu-like symptoms are sometimes reported for people easing off the drug).

One more related item: A physician might prescribe lidocaine patches. Lidocaine numbs tissue in the specific area where it is applied. They offer temporary relief without nasty side effects.

When it comes to prescription drugs, they usually work. But there are typically side effects. Follow instructions from a doctor and pharmacist.

Cost:

From inexpensive for generics, to expensive for name brands.

Bottom line:

I don't plan to take a prescription drug for pain unless I have surgery again. More risk of dependency than I'm willing to take. But they usually work to relieve pain.

8. Back Brace

You've seen people wear back braces, often by people who stand for long periods of time in their jobs. But some people wear them to manage back pain.

I'm not convinced they have helped me. Maybe it's because for it to be effective it needs to be snug or downright tight. It may help if muscles need support.

After my spinal fusion surgery, I wore a back brace for several weeks. But that situation was different: the brace was there because I had surgery and it was weeks of recovery.

But for spinal stenosis, the problem is that the nerves in the spine are already squeezed together and I don't want mine to be squeezed more!

So, the squeezing makes me worse.

I have a back brace that produces less "squeeze" and uses Velcro patches to secure a cold pack. It's one way to ice down the back. But I got tired of using it, due to the hassle of putting it on and the discomfort of wearing it. So it's gathering dust in my closet.

A really good back brace can be expensive. Before spending money to buy one, I suggest that you ask around and borrow one from a friend (chances are good that people you know will have one that's unused—if it's unused, that's your sign it didn't work for them).

Cost:

Anywhere from $20-$100 or more (but try borrowing one first).

Bottom Line:

You have little to lose when trying one, and maybe you'll be pleasantly surprised.

9. Walking

I'm a big advocate of walking, and I try to walk most days. The benefits of walking are numerous for good general health, but for back pain, it's usually when I've been in the most pain that it's been needed most to get my body moving again.

There's not much else that I can say about walking except to try it.

It costs nothing (except owning a good pair of walking shoes). There are dozens of pedometers or fitness trackers that will count your steps each day. Experts recommend that you walk 10,000 steps daily. That sounds like a huge number! And, well, it is.

Let's break it down: It's estimated the average person has a stride length of 2.1 to 2.5 feet. That means you'll take 2,000 steps to walk one mile. To get to 10,000 steps comes to five miles.

Wow. I'm tired just thinking about this! And I probably walk a mile or so most days ... making me wonder how I can possibly get to five miles.

For those of us with spinal stenosis, getting a couple of miles every day may be a tough challenge. So, no lectures from me on how much you should walk, except to say that I encourage you to walk as much as you can.

Cost:

Just good walking shoes!

Bottom line:

Walk as much as you can. It can benefit your health in so many ways beyond helping to loosen your back. Try to walk for 20 minutes. Work up to greater distances or lengths of time as your body allows.

10. Weight Lifting

I've never been a gym rat. I don't like lifting weights. It's just not my thing.

After my spinal fusion surgery, while in physical therapy the protocol was to lift weights to regain strength.

After my PT was over, I asked the therapists about lifting weights at the gym. They encouraged me to do so. And that's what I did regularly for about five years after the surgery.

But I've come to realize that lifting weights has probably aggravated my pain. Discussions with other healthcare providers suggest that weight resistance (lifting weights) isn't helpful for someone with spinal stenosis. But using your body's weight to strengthen muscles—particularly your core muscles—can be a positive thing to do.

So I guess it's a good thing I've never liked weight lifting, because I don't plan to take it up again.

Cost:

Monthly gym membership can run around $50+. Purchasing equipment for your home can start at $1,000 and up.

Bottom line:

Exercise is important, and lifting weights is normally a good thing to do for a healthy person. But for the individual with spinal stenosis, I can't recommend lifting weights. For me, weight lifting made my pain worse.

11. Stretching

I don't mind stretching. I just don't have the patience for it.

A lot of people have told me to do it, but sometimes I think it leaves me in more pain and I should just leave well enough alone.

I'm hardly a physician, but my theory is that the problem for a spinal stenosis sufferer is that it's not the muscles that are causing the problem. It's the narrowing of the nerves in the spine. The inferred pain is in the muscles. So stretching doesn't help my sore achy muscles, and it certainly isn't doing anything to help reverse the narrowing of the spine. Again, this is my theory and opinion only.

Sometimes, in the moment, the stretch feels good, but after I've stretched, I feel sore. So for me, stretching is not part of a spinal stenosis improvement plan.

Cost:

Nothing. Free videos on YouTube can show you some stretches to try for yourself. Or, get a book with illustrations. Or, ask a physical therapist or chiropractor.

Bottom line:

If you haven't tried stretching, you have little to lose by trying it for a few days. But if you find it gives you more pain, I'd suggest stopping it.

12. Swimming

I don't know how to swim. I just tread water and pretend. But I like being in water and doing what I can to swim. And I'll add water aerobics into the category of swimming.

Perhaps it's the buoyancy of the water that helps ease pain. Just walking around in a pool offers good resistance without aggravating the pain in my case.

If you engage in water aerobics, I do have a word of caution that you shouldn't overdo it, which means often not doing a lot of what the instructors say (I've found they don't care how much you do, just work out at your own pace). The instructors I've observed incorporate a lot of bouncing into the routine. For spinal stenosis, I don't think that's good. If there is already narrowing and the discs in the back are worn, hitting the bottom of the pool and jarring the back can't be good.

My monthly gym membership is well worth the cost just for access to year-round swimming and aerobics classes.

Cost:

Gym membership monthly can be around $50-and-up. Larger gyms with an indoor pool can command a higher monthly membership fee.

Bottom line:

Look into swimming and water aerobics ... but if you're in a lot of pain, go slowly. You may need to work up to it.

13. Chiropractic

I've gone to chiropractors for more than 40 years. And I continue to go at least once weekly. The right chiropractor helps me significantly. Being aligned takes away one element of pain for me. But I'm not sure spinal stenosis—the narrowing of the spaces within the spine—can be helped by chiropractic.

So to be clear: I go to a chiropractor weekly to make sure my body is properly aligned.

There's another aspect of chiropractic that I've come to learn over the years. Not all chiropractors will do this, but I suggest finding one who understands how to move the psoas muscle back into place. I'll address the psoas muscle more in the next section.

I've seen a lot of chiropractors over the years. Most are wonderful. I've experienced some who immediately want to put you through x-rays. Then they want you to come in three times a week for months. I'm skeptical of those because it seems to be way more treatment than is needed. Weekly adjustments? Yes. I encourage it.

Cost:

$50-$80 per adjustment. If you go weekly, this becomes $200 and more in monthly cost, unless you find a chiropractor or a chiropractic franchise with monthly memberships. Practices with memberships usually offer four adjustments in a month for under $100. If you can't find a practice with monthly memberships, have a conversation with your chiropractor and see if he or she would consider a monthly package to save you money.

Bottom line:

I believe in regular chiropractic adjustments—not so much for the spinal stenosis, but to alleviate other back pain that when added on top of stenosis, can make for very painful days.

14. Psoas Muscle Adjustments

"What is the psoas muscle?" you may wonder. It's a major, long muscle. Technically, it extends from the side of the lumbar region of the vertebral column and brim of the lessor pelvis. It joins the iliacus muscle to form the iliopsoas.

As a spinal stenosis sufferer, my layman's description is that it extends from the thigh, through the groin area, up into my abdomen. I've found in recent years that when a chiropractor (and other healthcare practitioners who know what they're doing) put pressure on my abdomen and move it back into place, that my low back pain subsides. As I become more in tune with my body, I can sense when it's off and is in need of adjustment.

Another option is to stretch the psoas muscle. You can go to YouTube and search for videos of how to do it.

Cost:

If a chiropractor incorporates this in an adjustment, then there shouldn't be an additional cost. I've also gone to massage therapists who know how to deal with the psoas muscle.

Bottom line:

Be informed and start to become intuitive about the psoas muscle and when it's in need of adjustment. When it's out of whack, find someone to move it back into place.

15. Kinesiology Taping

Kinesiology taping is popular among athletes, but a number of years ago I went to a chiropractor who had been trained (or perhaps self-taught) to apply tape.

KT, as it's called, was developed by a Japanese chiropractor in the 1970s, with the intention to alleviate pain and improve the healing in soft tissues. KT can be applied in the shape of a "Y," "I," "X," "Fan," "Web," or "Donut." The shape selection depends on the size of the affected muscle and the result desired.

If you do additional research, you'll read mixed reviews of its effectiveness. I think it gave me some relief, but admit I no longer do it (partly because I go to a different chiropractor these days).

As you might imagine, it's difficult, if not impossible, to tape yourself. You need someone who has been trained. Alternatively, watch YouTube videos for ideas.

Cost:

The taping I had done several years ago was from a chiropractor, and I wasn't charged an additional cost for the taping.

Bottom line:

It helped me several years ago, before my spinal stenosis diagnosis. If you can try it for no, or low cost, why not? You might be surprised with it offering some temporary relief.

16. Massage

If you've ever had a massage, you've probably enjoyed it. They can be relaxing. They can hurt a lot, too. Over the years, I've had many, many massages. A great massage helps me.

The key is finding someone who gives you a good massage with firm enough pressure to help relieve muscle stress, but who doesn't hurt you.

Some massage therapists give a relaxing massage (which doesn't involve deep tissue pressure). Others give sports massages which can be painful.

Rolfing (which I've tried) is painful. I'm sometimes a "no pain, no gain" guy, so I decided why not. It is an extremely painful massage that I tried for three months. Well, there was lots of pain, but after three months of weekly torture, I experienced no gain.

I've found that the benefits of a great massage will last me for a day or two, sometimes more. Like so many of the remedies you're reading here, massage can provide temporary relief. Over the years, I've averaged a massage at least twice monthly and, when I can afford it, weekly. The key is trying various techniques until you find a practitioner that you feel is most effective.

Cost:

$50-and-up for an hour.

Bottom line:

It may take trying a few massage therapists to find the person you like best, so don't base your evaluation of massage on just one person—or even a technique, unless you've experienced that technique from more than one masseur or masseuse.

17. Floatation Therapy

Floatation therapy enables your body to soak in magnesium sulfate (Epsom salt). You've probably heard, or experienced for yourself, how Epsom salt can reduce soreness.

I've experienced floatation therapy in a spa. Where I go, there is a private suite with a changing area and shower. You float undressed—although you can wear swimming gear if you wish—in a "float cabin." You might describe it as a shallow small pool (or oversized bathtub) with about a foot of water mixed with 800 pounds of Epsom salt.

Amazingly, the high salt content allows a person to float virtually effortlessly on top of the water. The Epsom salt acts as a muscle relaxer with anti-inflammatory properties. The water is 94 degrees, making it close to your body's temperature so it's comfortable.

After about an hour (longer if you book more time), the flotation therapy experience is over, but I've found that I really do feel relaxed and in less pain from having done it.

Cost:

An hour session at the location where I go is $80.

Bottom line:

It's a nice luxury that I like to do a few times yearly. I found it's relaxing and helps ease my pain temporarily.

18. Acupuncture

Back in the 1980s, I tried acupuncture. It did nothing for me. Fast forward to late 2016 when a friend encouraged me to go to her acupuncturist.

I've become a believer. I now love acupuncture, but I think it's vital to be performed by a master. My doctor is from China. He intuitively knows the practice and culture of acupuncture.

I began by taking a test before the first session so he could see the meridians that were blocked. Then I had 30-minutes of acupuncture on my lower back. I've been asked many times if the needles hurt. The sting was only slight. Once in a while an area will be hit where it takes a few seconds to adapt, but generally, I'd say there is no pain, just a split second of a modest sting that quickly goes away.

At my first session, I had difficulty even getting on the table. But when the 30 minutes were done and I sat up, I felt different. I can't say "better." Just "different."

Let's just say that I'm now a believer in acupuncture for spinal stenosis, pain management, and general wellness (it's even helped laryngitis). I can't explain it. Nor does it matter, as long as it offers relief. I should emphasize that I view acupuncture as pain management. I don't think it's a "cure" or a "fix." It's a tool to get you through one day at a time, or hopefully, one week to the next.

Cost:

My acupuncturist charges a one-year membership of $300. Each 30-minute session is then $50. Or, I can forego the membership and pay $80 per treatment. Surely, the cost of acupuncture will vary from one location to another.

I decided after my first session to commit to acupuncture daily for a couple of weeks, then three times weekly for a month, two times weekly for a couple of months, and now I'm at once (sometimes twice) a week.

You can do the math to see that in the first month I spent over $600, and now $200 or more monthly. I'd rather spend money elsewhere, as anyone would, but compare it to costly medical procedures and then decide what gives you the most relief.

Bottom line:

Most likely, I'll have weekly acupuncture for the rest of my life. That's how much I now believe in it.

19. Cryotherapy

I first read about cryotherapy a couple of years ago when providers started popping up in the area where I live, near Dallas, Texas. I was intrigued, but didn't look into it. Then one morning I woke up in worse pain than usual, and for unexplainable reasons I recalled the article I had read in the local newspaper, so decided to look into it.

A quick online search located two providers close to me. So I checked out one of them that same day. And am I glad that I did!

Cryotherapy is deep freezing. In this case, you stand inside a cylindrical chamber and the dry air inside is cooled by nitrogen to temperatures of anywhere from -250 to -300 degrees Fahrenheit. You're in the device for just three minutes and, for it to be effective, you'll need to completely undress (except keeping on socks ... and the facility I use provides mittens).

If you're like me, the prospect of being exposed to extreme cold temperatures doesn't sound inviting at all. But it's only three minutes. Surprisingly, it's not as cold as you might think. Where I go, there's an attendant with you the entire time to shut it off in less than the full three minutes if you can't tolerate it (the attendant only comes in after you're in the chamber, and you ring a doorbell to alert them to come in and start the device. They stay with you until the three minutes have passed before leaving the room).

When I first tried it, I purchased an unlimited pass for a month ($150). And I did get there nearly every day they were open, six days a week. So I definitely got my money's worth. Now I've backed down my visits to about once a week.

One other service provided by the cryotherapy place I use is the ability to get a spot treatment. So after I do the full-body freeze, sometimes I have three more minutes of extreme cold nitrogen blown onto my low back. It seems to knock out the inflammation for relief and it can last for several days for me.

Cost:

Surely it varies, but I buy a 10-pack for $150, making it $15 per visit. The spot treatment is an additional $10. Where I go, no appointment is necessary. It's walk-in and you take your turn. Wait times are short.

Bottom line:

Give it a try if you can. I realize for many people who may live in smaller cities or rural areas a cryotherapy center may not be close by. But I've observed that more and more places are opening around the country.

20. Whole Body Vibration

Whole body vibration (WBV) is a generic term used where any vibration of any frequency is transferred to the human body.

The Mayo Clinic says: *"Whole-body vibration can offer some fitness and health benefits, but it's not clear if it's as good for you as regular exercise. With whole-body vibration, you stand, sit or lie on a machine with a vibrating platform. As the machine vibrates, it transmits energy to your body, forcing your muscles to contract and relax dozens of times each second. The activity may cause you to feel as if you're exerting yourself. You may find a whole-body vibration machine at a local gym, or you can buy one for home use. Advocates say that as little as 15 minutes a day of whole-body vibration three times a week may aid weight loss, burn fat, improve flexibility, enhance blood flow, reduce muscle soreness after exercise, build strength and decrease the stress hormone cortisol. Some research shows that whole-body vibration, when performed correctly and under medical supervision when needed, can, reduce back pain, improve strength and balance in older adults, reduce bone loss."*

I first came across WBV at the cryotherapy center where I go to freeze. Their machines are among the higher-end technologies. I definitely felt different upon using it, and in the hours after using it the first time, could sense an improvement. But like many treatments, for the full benefit, it must be used frequently.

If you search "whole body vibration" you'll find many options for home purchase, and in a wide range of pricing.

This isn't for everyone. You need to be able to balance yourself while standing on the machine. But I like it.

Cost:

Wide range from a few hundred dollars to a few thousand dollars.

Bottom line:

I'd first see if there is a facility where you can test it. I've read that some manufacturers schedule demonstrations in retail stores. I suggest you try one before spending money to buy one. I like it, and plan to continue using it at the cryotherapy office I frequent.

21. Spinal Decompression

Spinal decompression is traction therapy. I describe it has having your upper body pulled away from your lower body to "decompress" the spine. Straps were placed around my chest and ankles to pull in opposite directions to stretch me out.

In theory, I thought it sounded like a great idea. But for me, it was painful. Really painful. As you read previously, I'm sometimes a "no pain, no gain" kinda guy, I figured I just needed to give it time to work. So I tried it again a couple of times.

The outcome after three visits was that it left me in greater pain than I was in prior to trying it. My Dad tried it, too, a few years ago. He stayed with it for weeks, yet found it to be of no help.

Of course, everyone is different. It might work for you. Knowing that many healthcare practitioners use spinal decompression, I have to assume it works for some people, just maybe not so well for those of us with spinal stenosis.

Cost:

Around $50 or more per session.

Bottom line:

I won't be trying it again.

22. Inversion Table

An inversion table is where you lean back on a table, and then it's flipped around so you're upside down. Your feet are higher than your head, stretching your back. In theory, it sounds good.

A massage therapist I had frequented had an inversion table and I tried it there. I found it very uncomfortable, mostly because of blood flow to the head. If you try it, make sure to do it on an empty stomach. I tried it only a handful of times, but I just didn't care for it, nor did I find it offered pain relief.

Cost:

If you purchase one, the costs vary greatly. I've seen them for as little as $100, but they can be much, much higher.

Bottom line:

I wouldn't purchase one, but if you have an opportunity to try it somewhere at little cost (or no cost), give it a shot. You never know until you try it at least once.

23. TENS Unit

I'm a fan of TENS (Transcutaneous Electrical Nerve Stimulation) units and have owned one for some time.

TENS is small battery-operated device for back pain treatment that uses low voltage electric current to relieve pain. The device can be hooked to a belt and is connected to two electrodes. It works by sending stimulating pulses across the surface of the skin and along the nerve strands. The stimulating pulses help prevent pain signals from reaching the brain. TENS devices also help stimulate your body to produce higher levels of endorphins, the body's natural painkillers.

My observation is that they give you "in the moment" pain relief. Perhaps it's because the pulses distract from pain. It's my observation that an hour after use that the pain slowly returns, hence why I suggest it's "in the moment" relief.

But that said, having temporary relief, even if only for a few minutes, can give your body and mind a break from the pain.

Cost:

You can buy them for as low as $30, but you can spend $100 or more.

Bottom line:

If you haven't tried a TENS unit, I try it, especially since they're relatively inexpensive and you can use them again and again.

24. Scenar Unit

What is a scenar? There are several types, but the one I use is the DOVE (Device Organizing Vital Energy) Scenar. The scenar uses low-frequency electrical stimulation (battery powered). If you search online for the DOVE Scenar, you'll read how it *"organizes and precisely focuses your body's bio-energy on fixing the problem."* It's also said that *"the DOVE scenar is an informational analogue of your body—a self-controlling and self-regulating system working on a FEEDBACK principle."* It doesn't hurt to use it, although if you turn up the frequency too high, it will sting. Here's more about it (copied from their website):

"The DOVE scenar is an adaptive electrical stimulator with a feedback feature. The device not only mimics the natural body language of electrical stimuli, but also constantly modifies them, based on real time feedback from the body. In other words, it "listens" to the body and enters into a dialog with it helping the body get its priorities straight. That's how it goes.

"Upon contact with the skin, The DOVE scenar sends an initial neuro-like electrical signal to the body (like saying, "Hello!"). The body registers the signal, recognizes it as "familiar" and responds to it (probably saying, "Don't you see, I am hurting here... Don't bug me"). The DOVE scenar reads the body response, modifies the next signal accordingly – and sends it back to the body telling it where to emphasize its healing efforts ("Hey, are you hurting HERE? Let's fix it together!").

"This exchange of information goes 60 times per second. On a chemical level, this dialogue excites the nervous fibers, especially B and C-type. These fibers, in turn, release floods of body's natural healing remedies and messenger molecules – neuro-peptides (or RP = Regulatory Peptides), locally to the site of the problem and into a bloodstream involving the entire body in the healing process.

"Basically, the DOVE scenar pushes the body to heal itself better and faster, by directing the body's attention, energy, and other resources to the site of a particular problem and by offering a friendly assistance in the process. The DOVE, however, leaves it up to the body to decide what it needs and wants to heal and in which order. This gives your body a unique chance to finally be heard and understood – as well as the chance to regulate its own treatment."

Cost:

The DOVE unit is expensive. Approaching $2,000.

Bottom line:

I use my scenar frequently. It goes with me whenever I travel. I feel the greatest relief when it's placed on my spine where it has narrowed. I hesitated about shelling out so much money, but have no regrets and would do it again. I also find it of help to reduce the pain of arthritis in my hand.

25. Over-the-Counter Pain Relief

As you read previously about my experience with NSAIDs (Nonsteroidal Anti-inflammatory Drugs), and how they ate holes in my stomach, I'm frightened of using them. Yet, some very popular name brands are NSAIDs, and I'll admit it: I use them from time to time. The difference, I suspect, is that the over-the-counter strength is much less than what I had been prescribed in 1990.

Still, I use OTC formulations sparingly. There are times when I've found the pain relief can take off the edge. My personal choices are Tylenol Arthritis Relief and Aleve. When the label says not to use them for more than a specified number of days, I adhere to it. Generally, I use these for only 2–3 consecutive days before backing off.

Cost:

Affordable.

Bottom line:

I use OTC pain relief as needed, and in moderation.

26. Pain Relief Supplements

You've probably had friends suggest certain pain relief supplements for pain (note: this is about pain relief supplements, not vitamins, minerals, or other dietary supplements you take for other reasons).

I have one I can recommend: Endocalyx™. It reduces inflammation. It works for me, and this is why I know it: I took it for several months in 2017 and 2018 and I was doing pretty well. Then in late 2018, I ran out and simply stopped taking it. My pain worsened. Upon restarting it, I sensed that I was better again.

There are many types of pain relief supplements. I glaze over thinking about them. Those I have tried have done nothing for me (except Endocalyx). I've come to realize that formulations in supplements are all over the place. What's inexpensive usually has a woefully inadequate dosage of ingredients (and it doesn't help to double or even triple the dose).

Coconut oil is believed to do a lot of good things for your health. I've used coconut oil off and on for years in my diet. I also understand that coconut oil can help relieve pain. I can't conclusively say that it does or doesn't.

Cost:

Widely varies.

Bottom line:

You have nothing to lose to try pain relief supplements, but if you don't think they are helping you, only you can decide if they're still worth it.

27. Food Sensitivity

Over the years I had often wondered if the food I was eating caused pain. You've probably heard of how gluten causes pain for some people. A close friend of mine has been off gluten for several years and has found some relief.

I decided to try a food sensitivity analysis that required a DNA saliva test combined with a blood test. Both specimens could be collected in my home. For the DNA test, you spit into a tube and mail it to a lab. For the blood test, the company sent all of the needed items where I pricked the side of an index finger and put small drops of blood on a special paper.

A few weeks later I got the results. For me, I have no foods that cause significant pain issues. But it's well documented that certain foods can aggravate pain.

Cost:

For the combined DNA and blood tests it was about $300.

Bottom line:

It only has to be done once. Even though the test didn't reveal anything for me, I'm glad that I did it. If you have any thoughts that food you're consuming may be contributing to pain, spending the money is a good way to get information. At least you will know what you can eat without it worrying about aggravating your pain.

28. Cannabidiol (CBD), Topical Creams, Lotions, and Potions

Today the rage is CBD Oil. I've tried three different types (there are so many it is dizzying). Honestly, I just didn't feel any different. I have tried a CBD topical cream. I think it helped. That said, I've heard and read where people say that CBD has changed their life, so as I've said before and I'll repeat: everyone is different.

My favorite topical ointments: Aspercreme® and a potion from my acupuncture doctor that's made in China called Hysan. Aspercreme and Hysan are just as good as CBD in my opinion, and a fraction of the cost.

I should also mention patches. You can buy them about anywhere. I also get herbal patches from my acupuncture doctor. It's temporary relief. The cost is so affordable that you should give them a try if you haven't already.

With any of these topical options, you just have to remember they won't "fix" the problem, but they do help, even if for only a few minutes or an hour to give you a short break from the pain.

Cost:

CBD products tend to be expensive. But most topical treatments, like Aspercreme, can be found at pharmacies and are affordable. The Hysan I referenced above can be found online, and it isn't very expensive.

Bottom line:

I don't let supplies of Aspercreme and Hysan get low at my house!

29. Ergonomics

There are ergonomic pens, keyboards, chairs, "thinger-grabbers" (okay, I don't know if that's a real term, but what I call a device to pick up my morning paper so I don't have to bend over) and more.

Like so many options, considering ergonomics is smart. As a writer, I use an ergonomic keyboard. I believe most of these devices are helpful, especially for the hands, neck, and upper back.

I haven't gone nuts at my house in converting everything, but where it makes sense, I seek out ergonomic-friendly devices.

Cost:

All over the map.

Bottom line:

Generally worth the investment.

30. Standing Desk

Even though I generally don't feel like standing and working, movement is occasionally needed. Using a standing desk can help. I have one where with the push of a button my desk goes up to my exact preferred height.

I should use my standing desk more often than I do. I can't comfortably stand for too long in any one place. But even a few minutes of standing (and working) can help.

I've seen all kinds of options for desks to enable a person to stand and work. Some involve a small stand you place on your desk. Others, like mine, are desks with a control switch so the desktop will go up in seconds by pushing a switch.

Cost:

Widely ranges from desk stands that are a few hundred dollars, all the way to the standing desk that is $2,000 and up.

Bottom line:

A standing desk is a luxury, due to the cost. But if you're at your desk a lot, it's worth it if you can afford it.

31. Handheld Spinal Traction Devices

There are multiple types of handheld spinal traction devices. You lay on the floor with your knees bent, and using the device you push on your thighs to stretch the low back. You push with as much pressure as you choose. For me, sometimes it helped; other times I think it hurt me.

When I read through the materials included with the device, it cautioned about using it if you've had any type of prior surgery. Well, I've had spinal fusion, so when I used it, I tried to be careful. But I've had enough times when I've felt that it hurt me so I've pretty much retired it to a place where it gathers dust.

But I don't blame the device. I think because of my surgery that it's simply not for me. As I've written previously, too, about the inversion tables and spinal decompression, I'm not convinced that stretching the spine for spinal stenosis sufferers is helpful.

Still, if you have back problems, and if you haven't had surgery, you might want to try it because it's a low cost possible solution.

Cost:

Around $40.

Bottom line:

Try it if you haven't had prior surgery. If you have had surgery in the past, you may want to steer clear of it. In any situation, read the instructions before use to see if there are any reasons you shouldn't use it.

32. Massage and Zero Gravity Chair

Another luxury: a massage chair. You've probably seen them in public places like shopping malls and airports. And you can buy them for your home.

My wife and I invested in both a massage chair and zero gravity chair (different than the inversion table described previously) for our 25th wedding anniversary.

The zero gravity chair is remarkably simple in design, but very comfortable. It tips you backward so that pressure is removed from your low back.

The massage chair is nice. It doesn't replace a massage by a trained professional, but it is relaxing in its own way. I love to sit in it to read the morning paper and drink coffee. I suggest 30 minutes as a maximum time to sit in it. It feels good in the moment, but generally doesn't offer relief beyond that.

Cost:

Widely ranges from $2,000 to $10,000 or more.

Bottom line:

I love my massage chair and zero gravity chair. But, there are really better and less expensive options for pain relief.

33. Mattress

The mattress you sleep on can make a difference, too. My wife and I have a Tempurpedic® bed. Because I'm so tall, we have a California King. It's been a good bed. But what I don't like about it is that because it's made of memory foam, with my size I slowly sink into the mattress over time and I've created an indentation in the mattress where my body lays.

I've had many friends highly recommend a Sleep Number® bed, which may be our next mattress purchase. With the ability to test firmness levels, surely there will be a better setting than others that will help. So while I can't say I've slept on a Sleep Number bed, it may be a good choice.

If you like your mattress, keep it! If you think it's giving you problems, I'd ask friends for their recommendations before shopping for a new one. Mattress comfort is a personal choice.

Cost:

A mattress is a sizeable investment, certainly hundreds, if not thousands of dollars.

Bottom line:

Since we spend around one-third of our lives sleeping on a mattress, you should get what you can afford, even if it stretches your budget.

34. Pillows

Sometimes I think sleeping hurts my entire body. So I'm a big believer in sleeping on a foam pillow that is form fitted for the neck and shoulders. When practical, I travel with it.

In addition to a pillow for my neck, I also use three additional pillows to relieve pressure for my back:

First, because I mostly sleep on my side, I place one king-size pillow between my legs to take pressure off of my low back. When I sleep on my back (which is infrequent) I place it under my knees.

The second pillow may be the most helpful. It's a formed leg pillow (you can search "formed leg pillow" and see several options). Even though a photo might show it in use positioned between the knees, I position it between my thighs. Since starting the use of this pillow, I think it's giving me relief.

Third, I place a regular sized pillow in front of me so that my arm rests on it to take pressure off my shoulder.

There are also full-size body pillows available. Because I'm extra tall, I'm not sure how they would work for me, hence my use of three pillows. But the people who I know who have full-size body pillows swear by them.

Cost:

For a quality pillow, you'll likely pay anywhere from $80 to $200.

Bottom line:

I recommend getting the right combination of pillows for better sleep, both for your neck, and your legs and shoulders. It may require trial and error, but given about a third of one's life is spent sleeping, experiment to see what works for you.

35. Hydration and Alkaline Water

I find my pain is worse when I don't drink enough water.

You've probably been told you should drink eight 8-ounce glasses of water a day. That's pretty close to what the Institute of Medicine suggests: 3 liters (13 cups) daily for men, and 2.2 liters (9 cups) daily for women. While all fluids count (coffee, etc.), I think the best course is to drink mostly water.

Second, I suggest including alkaline water when you can. Earlier, I wrote about going to cryotherapy, and one of the benefits where I go for my treatments is the bonus of a gallon of alkaline water every time I get frozen. They do it because research suggests that alkaline water can help reduce pain (using Scholar.Google.com, you can access authoritarian studies if you'd like to look into this topic more).

In my experience, I think there could be something to this statement. When I drink only alkaline water, I seem to have less pain. So do this: first, buy 2-3 gallons of alkaline water at your grocery store and drink it exclusively for 2-3 days and see if you feel a difference. Use it to make your coffee and tea, too. If you think it's helping, buy an alkaline water pitcher and filter.

Cost:

An alkaline water pitcher can be purchased online for under $40. A fully installed system can run hundreds, even thousands of dollars.

Bottom line:

I suggest buying bottled alkaline water for a few days to see if it's making a difference. If it is, consider buying an alkaline water pitcher and pitcher.

36. Meditation

I conclude this list with one thing that I have found helps me that doesn't involve potions, medical procedures, and the like.

It's meditation. I was introduced to someone who does meditation and energy work. I recognize that not everyone will buy into the concept of how the mind can influence how we respond to pain. My spinal stenosis and back pain is real, make no mistake. But when pause and give my mind quiet time, I can experience a few moments of less intense pain. Someone I spoke with suggested thinking and visualizing the area of pain as an energy field, and to isolate it and breathe it away. I do that. And I think it gives momentary relief, something I'm happy to take.

Cost:

You can conduct online research and get a lot of information free about meditation or spinning energy. Books on the topic of meditation abound. Or schedule an appointment with someone to experience it for yourself. Most are reasonably priced.

Bottom line:

I'll always meditate. I've found the benefits more than just helpful to relieving back pain.

Additional Options

Other options I haven't tried that I understand are expensive and aren't always covered by health insurance:

A. Stem Cell Therapy. I reviewed Platelet Rich Plasma (PRP) injections (#5), which is related to stem cell therapy. I'm a believer in PRP, and by extension, I suspect stem cell injections can be effective. If you explore either of these, I suggest taking Endocalyx (described in #36) for at least a month first to strengthen your microvascular system. Stem cell therapy is very expensive (I've heard $7,500 and up), but I've also heard from people have had had it done with success.

B. Spinal cord stimulation. In this case, the stimulator is surgically placed under the skin and sends a mild electric current to your spinal cord for pain relief.

C. Pulsed Electromagnetic Field. PEMF is widely used in Eastern Europe and other parts of Europe, where it has been a standard therapy. While this is a new technology in North America it is really an emerging technology.

D. Dry needling. It's also known as myofascial trigger point dry needling. It's the use of either solid filiform needles or hollow-core hypodermic needles for therapy of muscle pain, including pain related to myofascial pain syndrome. Dry needling is sometimes also known as intramuscular stimulation.

Summary

I estimate that I have to spend about an hour every day doing some sort of maintenance for my back.

And, as I wrote earlier, all of this costs hundreds of dollars monthly. Spinal stenosis has drained a lot of money away from day-to-day living and savings. As I see it, I can either invest the money in alternative procedures that help me so I can continue working and physically enjoy my life most days, or be miserable and not terribly productive most—if not all—days.

I've stated this before and I'll state it again: everyone is different. There is no "fix," in my opinion, only management of spinal stenosis. Try what makes sense for you. And good luck in finding the right combination of options that can offer you the most pain relief.

Made in United States
Orlando, FL
23 June 2023